You Got Sick— Now What?

Seven Secrets from Oriental Medicine to Eliminate the Cold and Flu

TOM INGEGNO
MSOM, LAc

iUniverse, Inc.
Bloomington

You Got Sick—Now What?
Seven Secrets from Oriental Medicine to Eliminate the Cold and Flu

The information, ideas, and suggestions in this book are not intended as a substitute for professional medical advice. Before following any suggestions contained in this book, you should consult your personal physician. Neither the author nor the publisher shall be liable or responsible for any loss or damage allegedly arising as a consequence of your use or application of any information or suggestions in this book.

iUniverse books may be ordered through booksellers or by contacting:

iUniverse
1663 Liberty Drive
Bloomington, IN 47403
www.iuniverse.com
1-800-Authors (1-800-288-4677)

Because of the dynamic nature of the Internet, any web addresses or links contained in this book may have changed since publication and may no longer be valid. The views expressed in this work are solely those of the author and do not necessarily reflect the views of the publisher, and the publisher hereby disclaims any responsibility for them.

Any people depicted in stock imagery provided by Thinkstock are models, and such images are being used for illustrative purposes only.

Certain stock imagery © Thinkstock.

ISBN: 978-1-4620-2334-9 (sc)
ISBN: 978-1-4620-2335-6 (ebk)

Library of Congress Control Number: 2011909645

Printed in the United States of America

iUniverse rev. date: 08/16/2011

CONTENTS

ACKNOWLEDGMENTS AND DEDICATION

To my wife and daughter for making my life so much more complete and my family for keeping me pointed in the right direction.

This book is dedicated to all the Oriental medicine practitioners, past and present, who have spanned several millennia and brought comfort to so many.

For all those ailing in the world,
Until their every sickness has been healed,
May I myself become for them
The doctor, nurse, the medicine itself.

—*Shantideva,* The Way of the Bodhisattva
Chapter 3, Verse 8

PREFACE

It seems as if somewhere along the way, we have forgotten to take care of ourselves. We quickly grab over-the-counter drugs to alleviate the symptoms of a cold or flu: coughs, congestion, aches, pains, chills, and fevers. We line up every flu season to get a shot, which is the medical community's best guess at what the next flu strains might be. This shot has even been linked to causing flu-like symptoms in adults. Being a true holistic practitioner, I am not saying that these modern remedies are unsafe or ineffective, but what if you took control of your health using some safe and effective traditional cures to eliminate—or at least shorten —the course and alleviate the symptoms of cold-weather diseases? The best part is that most of these cures can be applied quickly with little to no cost, and if the ailment is caught early enough, you can knock it out before your nose even has a chance to stuff up!

Today, no one can write a book offering advice on any topic, let alone health care, without writing a lengthy disclaimer, absolving the author of any and all responsibility when it comes to what the reader does with the information. As such, here is mine:

As with any health and wellness therapy, it is important to discuss these modalities with your physician (although most acupuncturists, chiropractors, naturopaths, and massage therapists may be well versed in these techniques) prior to administering them at home. These methods are extremely safe if practiced using good technique and common sense. This means if these techniques cause any pain, discomfort, or worsening of symptoms, stop immediately and consult your primary care physician. These techniques may not be appropriate for children under the age of twelve as fevers tend to spike very quickly into a dangerous range. Also, if you have an extremely high fever (104° F or higher) or have a fever lasting for more than three days, seek immediate medical attention.

Now that we have gotten that out of the way, read on!

Yours in Wellness,

Tom Ingegno, MSOM, LAc
Master of Science in Oriental Medicine
Licensed Acupuncturist (NY & MD)
Diplomat in Acupuncture (NCCAOM)

CHAPTER 1
The Scariest Thing in the World …
If It Happens to Be a Slow News Week

It seems like just yesterday everyone was panicking about the avian flu. We braced ourselves for the worst pandemic in the history of the world. Chickens were slaughtered and burned *en masse* to prevent the spread of the disease. People were quarantined, and the media made us afraid to leave our houses. My mother-in-law even convinced my wife to buy Tamiflu from one of those less-than-reputable Internet pharmacies. Although there were some outbreaks around the world in small, isolated cases, after all was said and done, few people actually ever contracted this flu, and even fewer died from it. Now we have the swine flu (also known as H1N1) rearing its ugly head, and although scientists, doctors, and health care workers alike are saying it's milder than the regular flu, good old H1N1 is getting more coverage than the O. J. Simpson case did. Why is there all this chaos for something that happens every season? Chances are it has been a slow news week.

I have been working in the field of Oriental medicine for over a decade, and it amazes me that people will cancel their acupuncture appointments when they are sick. Ask any acupuncturist or Oriental medicine practitioner, and he or she will tell you that when you are ill is when you need treatment the most. It seems that most of these patients were genuinely concerned for the well-being of others and did not wish to spread their germs to them. Although very thoughtful, it did leave them isolated at home for about a week without any palliative care.

It is the intention of this book to introduce Western individuals to some basic tools from traditional Asian healing modalities that will help reduce the duration of their symptoms. Most of these techniques are considered folk medicine in Asia and are frequently reached for at the first signs of a cold or flu, and are definitely used prior to going to the doctor. Hopefully this will provide you with some relief and shorten your self-quarantine.

Most of these remedies are so old, scholars often argue about their origins. These techniques and concepts have never gone out of style because they focus on helping the body overcome the disease instead of focusing on attacking the disease directly. This means that no matter what strain of a new virus or bacteria hits you, these remedies should help provide an easing of symptoms and a shorter duration of the ailment.

In each of the following chapters, a modality will be introduced that has been time tested for thousands of years. I have made attempts to deliver the safest and simplest techniques that still are effective. The chapters are in ascending order of difficulty of technique and can be used in conjunction with most of the other techniques. You will also find that certain therapies are even more effective when paired with others, but most therapies can be done on their own. You may use these techniques in conjunction with modern medicine, including prescriptions from your doctor or over-the-counter remedies. It is also safe to use other holistic modalities, such as healing touch, herbal medicine, and homeopathy, if you feel they are appropriate. If you consult an Oriental medical practitioner, the practitioner may have a different opinion about some of the techniques, but please keep in mind that this information is designed to be safe for all people who use it properly, and with nearly six thousand years of knowledge coming from all over Asia, techniques and theories differ widely depending on their particular school of thought and training.

Try these techniques and listen to yourself. Remember which ones work best and use them the second you feel like you are catching a cold or the flu. You may be able to bypass the entire course of illness.

CHAPTER 2
Heat Therapy: Sweating It Out

I'm not sure if there is any fact to the old adage "Starve a fever, feed a cold," but I do know one true biological fact that is not as catchy but is of much greater use. That fact is that organisms live and function most efficiently closer to the upper range of their temperature threshold. What this means is that bacteria, viruses, cows, otters, and humans all function and have a better ability to survive on the warmer side of their temperature limits.

For example, let's say you were stranded on a desert island with unlimited food and water, but no fire, no shelter, and no real way for you to regulate your temperature externally. If it were a constant 85 degrees outside, you could survive nicely with no real problems. If the temperature went up to 110 degrees and there was no way to cool yourself down, chances are you would eventually overheat and die, a mere 25 degrees hotter. Now if the temperature dropped from 85 degrees to 60 degrees, 50 degrees, or 40 degrees, you would be cold, but your body would eventually adjust, and while functions like metabolism would slow, you would still be able to function.

This example is true for most organisms, and the temperature range is much narrower for single-celled bacteria and viruses. Microbiologists exploit this fact all the time by cooling these simple organisms down to a state of near-suspended animation. How do they kill them? Well, other than harsh chemicals, heat does the trick nicely.

What does any of this have to do with how you can beat the cold and flu with heat? Your body naturally knows the answer. When we get a fever, it is not a symptom of the infection causing your body temperature to rise, but rather your body making it harder for the infecting organism to work. It is literally trying to burn out its attacker. Sometimes our body pushes things too far, and we can have complications from the fever; this is clearly the time for medical intervention, especially in children and the immunodeficient, but in most cases the body knows exactly how far to push.

Oriental medicine compares the skin to a battleground between your immune system, referred to as wei qi (way chee), and the invading pathogen. The skin is a physical barrier that helps keep the enemy out. In fact, both Eastern and Western medicine acknowledge the skin as the largest immune system organ in the body. As the enemy pushes in and advances, we may get chills. When the wei qi is winning, we start to feel hot and get feverish. When the pores open and we begin to sweat, the theory is that our wei qi has won the battle, and along with the sweat, the invading pathogen is being driven out. From a Western standpoint, when the fever breaks, we sweat, start feeling better, and are on the road to recovery.

This is the easiest of all techniques to do because it requires very little effort on your part, which is especially nice when you are feeling under the weather, and can be accomplished several different ways. Please feel free to do any or all of them.

1. One of the best methods is vigorous exercise. As you work out, you increase circulation, which helps pump white blood cells to the infection. This process will help carry away metabolic waste, raise your internal body temperature, and most importantly, make you sweat! I understand that with body aches, congestion, headaches, and chills, you might not feel up to moving much, but if you can get moving, you will feel better, at least for the amount of time you are working out. Your preferred workout method is okay, but remember not to push yourself too hard. This is not a workout to max your body out, but it's just to get things moving and warmed up. Please check out the qigong chapter for some gentle exercises to help you boost your immune system and heat up at the same time.

2. The next method I would like to talk about is the easiest and my favorite. That being said, you will probably get

some weird looks in your household. When you start to feel ill, pull out your cold-weather clothes. Yes, put on your warmest sweater, hat, scarf, sweat pants, wool socks, and jacket, and get under some blankets. You will eventually start to feel hot. This is good. Stay under these layers until you have a good solid sweat going.

3. This suggestion works very well with bundling up. Increase your intake of hot liquids. Tea and soup are great. Chicken soup has been shown to have immune-boosting functions, so why not use it? Oriental medicine would look not only at the temperature but also at the spiciness of the food. Some Oriental "cold and flu" soup recipes will be given in the next chapter, but remember, you can always add a bit of hot sauce or red pepper flakes.

4. Hot showers and baths can be used to help open the pores as well. You might not notice if you are sweating, but the added heat will help drive out the pathogens. In Japan, many people soak in hot springs with temperatures as high a 107°. That is good, but it is also very hot. Temperatures between 102 and 106 will do just fine. Spend at least twenty minutes in water this warm and try to keep as much of your body submerged as possible. If at all possible, try and get the back of your neck underwater as well. There are several acupuncture points in this area that open directly to the inside of your body. This is why even on mild days you may see Chinese people wearing a scarf; they are covering this area to keep out pathogens. If you are also sore and achy, feel free to add 1/4 cup of Epsom salt to the bath. If you have a stuffy nose, add a few drops of essential oils, like eucalyptus or peppermint. The most important thing here is that you are helping your wei qi heat the body to drive out the pathogen.

Feel free to combine any or all of these methods with the methods discussed in the next chapters. *Please note that if your body temperature goes higher than 104 °F without sweating or the fever does not break within a few days, you need medical attention!*

CHAPTER 3
Soups: Simple, Tasty, Effective

If you have your favorite recipe passed down from your grandmother, please use it. Comfort may help ease the symptoms of a cold or flu all by itself. Here are some basic recipes to add into rotation to help you bounce back to health. I have chosen a few simple recipes, because the ingredients are easy to obtain, they taste good, and they are quick to make. There are thousands of soup recipes that can be useful to treat a cold. Simple additions to your favorite recipe may boost the health benefits for you.

Nearly everyone has a favorite chicken soup recipe, and health benefits have actually been found to back up the claims that chicken soup actually does support immune system function. When people call it Jewish penicillin,[1] there is some real truth to that. If you have a favorite recipe, try adding any or all of the following ingredients to taste. Spices like *cinnamon* and *hot pepper* add heat to your system and help you sweat. If you have a favorite hot sauce, go ahead and add a few drops to your soup. It will have the same properties as the hot pepper and may actually help clear your sinuses as well! *Licorice root* (not the candy) can be added to help soothe a sore throat and has the properties of smoothing the qi flow throughout the acupuncture channels. One of the major theories of Oriental medicine is that when disease is present in the body, the qi (life energy) doesn't circulate smoothly. Licorice is said to harmonize the channels and help the qi return to a normal flow. *Onions, scallions,* and *garlic* all have been shown to boost immune system function and have been praised for their antibacterial and antiviral properties. In Chinese herbal medicine, these are said to help open the orifices and drive out pathogens. *Mushrooms*, especially reishi, miitake, and shitake, have been shown to have high levels of polysaccharides and amino acids that strongly stimulate immune system function.[2]

It might be a good idea to avoid the following soups when you are sick:

- *Any soup that has dairy in it.* Dairy produces mucus, as a result of the amino acid found in milk (specifically cow's milk) called casein. Casein is extremely sticky. In fact, many white glues use this compound as the main ingredient. Have you ever wondered why there is a cow on the front of a very popular type of glue? Casein, when ingested by most humans, cannot be broken down easily, which can be a problem even for those who are not lactose intolerant. The compound binds to most surfaces in the body, especially the mucous membranes, making an already unpleasant situation much worse. On a side note, many holistic nutritionists say to eliminate dairy completely from one's diet. Besides increased mucous production, dairy products have been linked to arthritis and several gastrointestinal disorders.

- *Cold soups.* Many of you would instinctively cringe at the thought of a cup of cold gazpacho while you are suffering with the chills, fever, throbbing head and all the other symptoms that make up a cold or flu. It's a good idea to avoid them just in case. Cold soups will lower your core body temperature, counteracting what your body is trying to do with the fever.

- *Thick, heavy soups or stews.* Putting heavy foods into your system when you feel sick probably also seems unappealing, but some people may feel the need to eat something heavy in an attempt to give the body more energy to fight the cold. This isn't a bad theory, but in practice it further taxes the digestive system because it makes those nutrients harder to absorb. Soups that have a thin broth are more easily absorbed during illness and also provide you with additional fluids to keep you hydrated and help flush out any metabolic waste from fighting your illness.

In the Chinese language, the word for soup is *tang*. This word not only means a soup that you would eat for the simple enjoyment of food, but also an herbal decoction, including teas. The use of this word points out a strong connection to the theory that food is medicine. In fact, Chinese five spice powder, a common spice mixture used in Chinese cooking, is said to balance out the five elements of the body. Without getting into a lengthy discussion about Oriental medical theory, the five elements of the body are fire, earth, metal, water, and wood. Each of these elements has particular functions, energy pathways, and organs they influence, and they each even have tastes and smells. When a person is healthy, these five elements function in unison; when illness sets in, one of these elements gets too strong or too weak, throwing the energy systems out of balance. The Chinese five spice powder was meant not only to hit the five different tastes, but also to harmonize the energetics of the food, making a simple meal even more nutritious.

The next few pages include some simple soup recipes; please feel free to modify them slightly to suit your tastes. With all of these recipes, it is strongly suggested that while drinking them, you bundle up and remain that way until you break a sweat.

Simple Chai Tea

Technically, this is not a soup, but it does have several aromatic herbs in it that provide an added boost to help you recover from a cold. Chai tea has an interesting history. It was really a marriage between Indian teas, which usually included herbs and spices, and a proper British black tea. It evolved sometime during the British occupation of India, when milk was added to a traditional Indian herbal tea.[3] As stated before, avoid milk because it produces phlegm. Try adding soy milk instead. There are thousands of chai recipes available, and herbs can be omitted or added as you see fit. Most traditional blends take quite a bit of time to prepare. This may not be completely traditional, but we are looking for a more therapeutic effect.

> Ingredients:
>   3 thumbnail-sized slices of fresh ginger about ¼-inch thick
>   1 cinnamon stick
>   3 cloves
>   3 cardamom pods (or 4 seeds)
>   3 black pepper seeds
>   2 teaspoons of a good black tea, preferably an Indian blend like Darjeeling. You can also use 2 tea bags for ease

Take the cinnamon, cardamom, cloves, and black pepper, and crack them up, either by using a mortar and pestle or by placing the ingredients in a bag and hitting them with a spoon. This will release some of the oils and will provide a stronger flavor. If you do this too far in advance, say a day or two, these oils will dissipate and you will lose both the flavor and the therapeutic effect.

Bring 2 cups of water to a boil and add the crushed herbs and ginger. Reduce the heat to a simmer for about 5 minutes.

Add the tea and let it steep for another 5 minutes.

Strain into a mug and add sugar or honey to taste.

*** If you were to add milk, it can be added after the tea and allowed to simmer for a few minutes. ***

All these aromatics are said to open the sinuses as well as warm the body. Hopefully, drinking this will help open pores and make you break a sweat.

Today many people make chai tea with green, oolong, white, or red tea. Black tea is considered to be the "warmest" of teas, according to Oriental medicinal principles on food. It is said that the preparation process, namely drying and fermenting the tea, adds a warming property to it.[4] Teas that are not fermented—such as green, white, and most herbal teas, as well as oolong, which is partially fermented—are cooler in comparison. To get the most "heat" into the chai tea, black tea is suggested, but if you dislike the taste or wish to avoid the caffeine, you can substitute another type of tea.

Ginger and Scallion Soup

Here's a very simple recipe. The two main ingredients will open the orifices (sinus and nasal passages) and warm the interior. It is an extremely light broth and can be drunk throughout the duration of your illness.

Ingredients:
2–3 scallions chopped, both the white and green parts
3–5 thumbnail-size pieces of ginger about ¼ " thick
1–2 cloves of garlic minced
Salt to taste
Black pepper to taste

Take 4 cups of water or chicken broth and add ingredients. Bring to a boil and reduce heat. Simmer until about 3 cups are left. Bundle up and drink 1 cup every half hour until sweating begins.

Gui Zhi Tang (Cinnamon Twig Formula)

Classically, this formula is used for conditions in Oriental medicine called internal cold, referring to diseases that make your body feel cold on the inside. It is extremely safe to use because most of these herbs are common food items. This soup is more of a Chinese herbal formula.[5] You might want to have a discussion with your acupuncturist or herbalist on the many herbal formulas used to treat the cold and flu. The wide variety of formulas for these conditions work best at the first sign of a cold. The entire scope of herbal medicine for the cold and flu would be too great for the contents of this book, and for the sake of simplicity, this formula will be the only one included.

> 9 g Gui Zhi (cinnamon twig)[6]
> 9 g Bai Shao Yao (peony root)[7]
> 9 g Sheng Jiang (fresh ginger)
> 12 Dao Zao (Chinese dates)
> 6 g Zhi Gan Cao (honey-fried licorice root)

These herbs are fairly common in Asian grocery stores and can definitely be found online. There are many prepared pill versions of this formula, but having it warm on hand adds a bit more heat to the mix. This formula is prepared by placing all the herbs in a pot with 4 cups of water. Bring the herbs to a boil and simmer until there are approximately 3 cups left. Strain the liquid and drink 1 cup three times per day. This can be repeated for three days or until the fever has broken.

Please note that licorice (the herb, not the candy) has been shown to raise blood pressure slightly.[8] If you have high blood pressure or are taking medication for your blood pressure, avoid this formula.

CHAPTER 4
Qigong and Other Weird Terms for Breathing

When you say terms like *qigong* (pronounced chee kung) or explain breathing exercises to someone who is not familiar with these terms, you are bound to get some odd looks. In the last twenty years, Americans have started to embrace tai chi, the relaxing and slow-paced martial art, because of its many health benefits. Tai chi itself is a form of qigong. A simple explanation of qigong is a series of gentle movements coordinated with the breath to help promote health. It is theorized that the body has pathways called meridians. These meridians bring qi, or energy, to nourish all tissue. When we are sick, it is believed that the qi is either too weak or stuck in a location where illness can set in. Qigong is used to help strengthen the qi as well as smooth the flow through the meridians, thus helping your body recover.

This chapter will cover the some basic breathing techniques and some qigong and breathing exercises to help build your qi and expel your cold or flu. These are great because they not only get you breathing and moving, they also help you break a sweat (as suggested in a previous chapter). If possible, do some of these exercises when you are feeling healthy, especially the basic breathing, as it will keep your immune system running optimally and could possibly help you avoid the cold altogether. Please understand that there are thousands of qigong, yoga, and breathing exercises that may be helpful during the cold and flu. This book is concentrating on the simplest ones so the techniques can quickly be put into practice. If you would like more information on any of these arts, please consult a well-qualified teacher.

A note of caution: if any of these exercises make you light-headed or uncomfortable, stop immediately and sit or lie down if necessary. Do not overdo them. At all times, they should feel comfortable and relaxing.

Basic Breathing

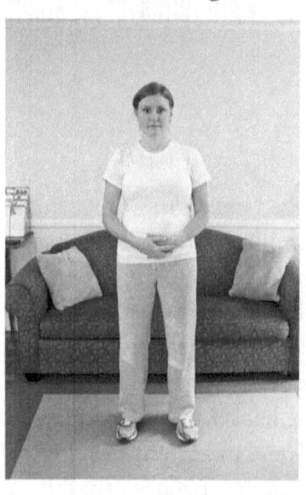

I once saw Dr. Andrew Weil on a talk show and he attributed many of our illnesses to not breathing properly. Many of the stress-related problems we have could be easily helped by taking the time to breathe. When we are stressed, our immune system does not function as well as it could, and we can become sick. While breathing techniques are widely taught in qigong, meditation, and yoga classes, simple techniques can be done at home or work in just a few short minutes. The following technique can help relieve stress, relax the body, and clear the mind. Use this technique wherever you are and at any time to achieve some peace in your life. If used prior to a cold, it will tonify your immune system. This breathing exercise has been included because it is a precursor for all other techniques and is an easy entry point into all the other breathing exercises. If you are suffering from a cold or the flu, you might be having problems breathing in and out of your nose. This is okay; practice the abdominal breathing in an out of the mouth and you may find that your sinuses open at least briefly while doing the exercise.

1. Find a comfortable position. It can be sitting, standing, or lying down. Soften or close your eyes.

2. Place your hands directly below your belly button.

3. Slowly inhale through the nose if possible. If this is not possible, breathe through your mouth. If your sinuses

open up, switch to breathing through the nose. Try filling the area under your hands. Do not force air in; try only to allow the abdomen to expand as far as comfortable. If it helps, imagine the air going into the belly and expanding. This should be relaxed and not forced; keep the breathing as quiet and natural as possible.

4. Exhale slowly through the mouth, allowing the abdomen to contract naturally.

5. Repeat for at least ten breaths or until you feel more relaxed. It might be difficult to do too many of these, but try ten before you decide to do more. As always, listen to your body.

6. Try this several times a day when you are sick. Getting more oxygen into your body will give you more energy and help boost your immune system function.

This technique is often referred to as "Infant Breathing" because it mirrors the way a baby's belly rises and falls with each breath. Pay attention to your ribs and shoulders; they should only move slightly and the sensation should be that you are drawing air deep into your abdomen.

Hold Ball

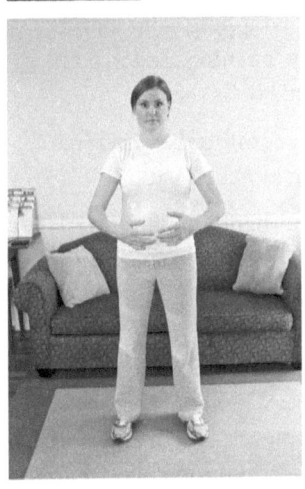

For this technique, you will follow the same breathing guidelines as the basic breathing described previously. This technique is said to tonify qi, and many report feeling warmer all over. People also experience tingling, heaviness in the hands, and in general feel better than they did before the exercise. It seems to have a strong resonance with the spleen and stomach meridians, which in Oriental medicine take in food nutrients and help convert it into blood and qi, which are the building blocks for all functions throughout the body. Here's how to perform the technique:

1. Stand in a comfortable position with your feet shoulder-width apart. Relax your shoulders and allow your hands to fall naturally at your sides. There should be a small space between the arm and the side of the body, as if you were holding an egg under the armpits. Knees should be straight but not locked. People wishing for a heavier "workout" can bend their knees so it looks as if they are sitting on a high stool.

2. Gently tuck your chin and imagine a string from the crown of your head pulling upward.

3. Curve your hips forward and allow your back to straighten. To practice this, you can stand with your back against a wall and try to make as much of the spine as possible touch the wall. Perfectly straight is not the goal, just straight and relaxed. This should be a comfortable position.

4. Begin the basic breath. As stated before, try breathing in through the nose and out through the mouth, but make adjustments as needed if you are congested.

5. When you are ready, inhale and allow the palms to raise up with fingertips facing each other, level with the navel. Extend your arms as if you were wrapping your hands around a tree. There should be an opening under your armpits as if you were holding tennis balls there.

6. Hold this position for as long as it is comfortable. Feel free to adjust the breathing and posture as necessary.

7. Finish on an exhale and allow the hands to float back down to your sides. Take a few more breaths and move around or shake out as you see fit.

The Hold Ball technique is said to help harmonize the spleen and stomach systems and leave you feeling stronger with more energy to fight off illness. This is important because regulating the spleen and stomach energy helps your body have enough energy to fight off colds.

Fire Circle

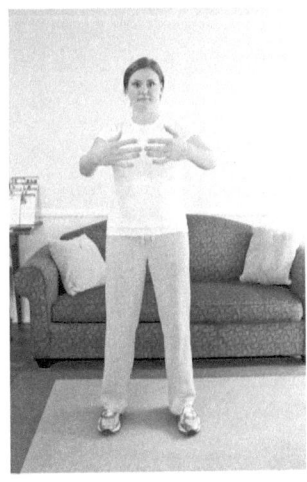

As the name implies, this might make you a bit warmer. The fire element is associated with the heart in Oriental medicine, and this position will be similar to the last exercise, with your hands held higher and level with the heart.

1. You may start this exercise from:
   a) the Hold Ball position
   b) the basic standing position with feet shoulder-width apart; shoulders relaxed, back, and down; arms hanging comfortably at sides; knees slightly bent; and chin slightly tucked.

2. With the inhale, bring your hands up slowly, level with your sternum.

3. Imagine your are holding a wagon wheel in your arms, keeping them as round as possible without being uncomfortable.

4. The tips of the fingers from each side should be pointing at each other with whatever distance is comfortable for you between them.

5. Your gaze can be at the palms of the hands or softened and looking out between the space between your two middle fingers.

6. Continue inhaling through the nose (if possible) and out through the mouth.

7. You may imagine that you heart is a roaring fire, and as it burns, your body feels warmer.

8. You may also imagine that fire is spreading out and connecting the circle that is your arms.

9. Hold and continue breathing for as long as it is comfortable.

10. When you are done with the exercise, slowly lower your hands down to your sides as you exhale.

11. Take a few cleansing breaths and shake out or move around as you see fit.

This is a technique often used to help people improve circulation and warm up. Combined with the Hold Ball position, many people may be able to break a sweat easily. Remember, breaking a sweat means we are winning the battle against our invading pathogen.

Breath of Fire

This breathing is traditionally from a branch of yoga called Kundalini. The Kundalini system is designed to help stimulate the energy flow from the base of the spine to the crown of the head. Breath of fire, or *agni-prasana* in Sanskrit, can be done as a stand-alone exercise or with other yoga exercises. This is a more advanced breathing technique and will take some time to feel comfortable. Practice short rounds of thirty seconds or so until the breath feels more natural. Be careful: some people may get light-headed with this technique. If your sinuses are very congested, this technique may not work for you. Try doing some of the other exercises and see if your congestion clears before attempting this breath.

1. Find a comfortable standing, seated, or lying down position.

2. Start doing some deep, relaxed abdominal breathing as described in the basic breathing technique.

3. When ready, exhale with a short forceful breath out of the nose. This is achieved by pulling the abdominal muscles in.

4. The inhale should be relaxed and last two to three seconds, followed by another short forceful exhale.

5. Repeat this exercise for thirty seconds to two minutes for as long as it is comfortable.

This technique can be done several times a day and is great for a quick boost of energy when you are feeling run down. This is precisely the reason it has been included in this text.

Wringing Out the Sponge

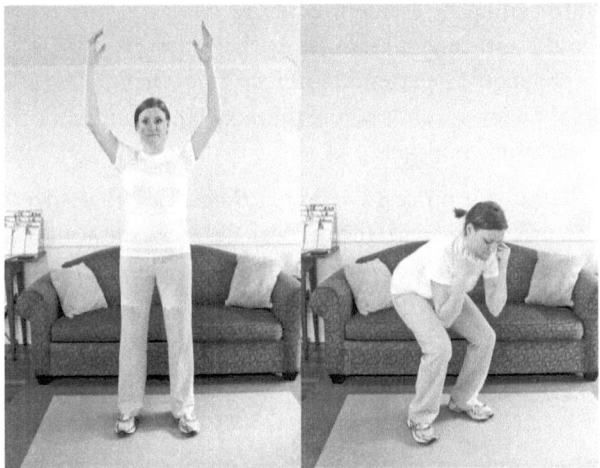

This qigong exercise requires more movement than the other techniques, and while it is a great exercise, it may be too strenuous for some people suffering with cold and flu symptoms. There are several variations on this exercise, and many people like to do this outside, facing the sun. If weather permits and you feel up to it, you should try to do this method outside as well. In this technique, you are visualizing yourself as a sponge that is full and needs to be wrung out. As you exhale, visualize the "dirt" of symptoms leaving your body, and during the inhale, you should visualize healing light filling up your body.

1. Start standing with feet about shoulder-width apart.

2. Do several basic breaths to prepare.

3. Inhale and raise your hands up as if reaching for the sun on the horizon.

4. As you exhale, slowly start to curl your body up as if squeezing out any illness. Your arms should pull down and curl into the chest while making a fist. Your back should arch slightly while you bring your chin to your chest. Your knees should bend down to a squat as low as is comfortable. Every muscle should tense and hold for a few seconds.

5. As you inhale, the muscles should relax as you expand, imagining the sunlight entering every cell of your body and nourishing all tissues. At the end of the inhale, your arms should be extended back up as if reaching for the sun. Take a few seconds before the next exhale and feel the sun warming your core.

6. Repeat this process five to ten times. End the process on an inhale, and with the next exhale, allow the arms to float down to your sides. Take a few moments and return to basic breathing before you end your breathing practice.

CHAPTER 5
Gua Sha: Scraping Away Evil Wetness (Two-Person Technique)

Gua sha sounds much weirder than it actually is. It roughly translates to "scraping away evil wetness," but it looks more like a massage being done with a tool. What kind of tool? Most Chinese will use a jar lid, a large coin, or an Asian-style soup spoon. They do sell fancy tools that are made out of jade or ox horn, but from experience, the spoon or metal jar lid work just as well. Gua sha can be done all over the body, but for cold and flu symptoms, it is most commonly applied to the neck

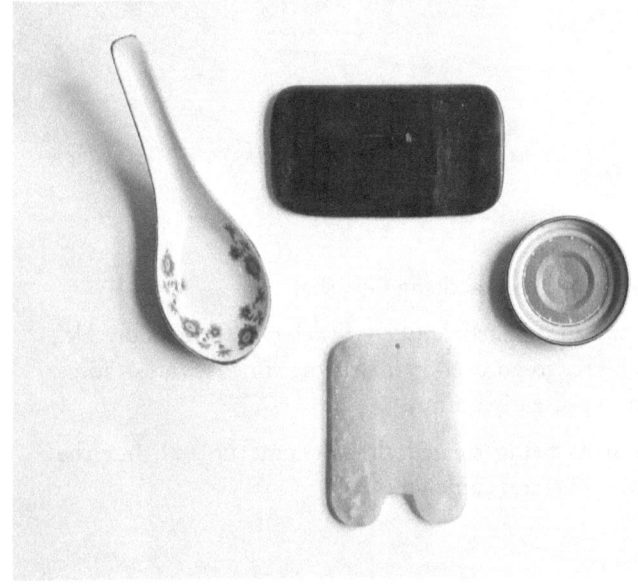

and back and in most cases done without oil or cream. For people suffering from cold and flu symptoms, sometimes a small amount of Vicks VapoRub may be applied to the neck, back, and chest before performing the technique.

Whichever tool is chosen should be held so that a rounded edge can gently scrape the surface of the skin with long strokes. The process is done until the skin develops a deep red color. Often, small purple or dark red spots called petechiae appear on the surface of the skin. These dots are a good sign and indicate that you can move to another area. The redness and spots may last up to a few days. The Oriental medical theory states that pathogenic factors like wind, heat, cold, dryness, and dampness can invade the body and cause disease. This disease fights with the wei qi (defensive energy, discussed in the heat therapy chapter) and can camp out below the surface of the skin. Scraping along the surface of the skin stimulates the wei qi, increases circulation of blood to the surface, and helps drive the pathogens out of the body. You will need someone to perform this technique on you, as it will mainly cover the back of the neck, shoulders, and area between the shoulder blades.

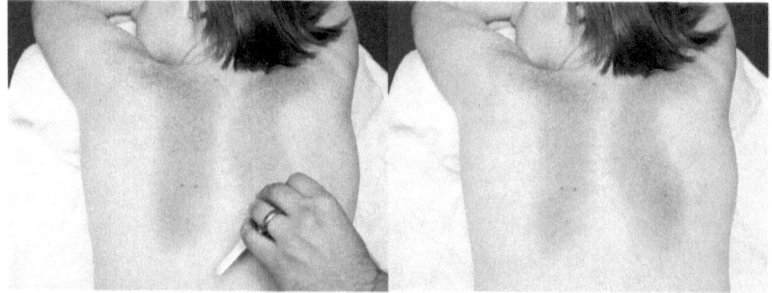

Some general tips when practicing Gua sha:

- The pressure applied should be firm but not uncomfortable. It is better to go over an area more times with less force than to cause discomfort.

- The areas being treated should come up red, but the redness may not come up evenly.

- If there is any bruising, blood, or discomfort, stop immediately! The person performing the technique could have been a little overzealous.

- Develop a stroke length and rhythm that is comfortable for the person being treated.

- The technique can be repeated after a few days when most of the redness clears.

Here's how to apply this technique:

1. The person performing the technique should hold the tool comfortably in his hand.

2. Starting with the base of the head, where the hairline ends, work down and outward, using long, even strokes toward the shoulder. Work on one side of the neck and shoulder until the area develops a deep red color.

3. Repeat on the other side of the neck. Working on this area can reduce fevers, open the sinuses, and relieve headaches.

4. Now, starting where the neck meets the shoulders, work straight down the back until you get to near the bottom of the ribs. Be careful not to hit the spine, as it may be painful to the patient. Stay on one side of the spine, but feel free to cover the whole muscle.

5. When one side of the back comes up red, move to the other side and repeat the process. Working this area stimulates the immune system, helps with coughs and congestion, and relieves body aches.

After receiving this treatment, the area may be warm or you may break into a sweat. Keep yourself covered and warm.

CHAPTER 6
Cupping: Not as Bad As it Sounds
(Two-Person Technique)

When Gwyneth Paltrow showed up to a movie premiere in a backless dress covered in perfectly circular bruises, cupping made its way into the spotlight. It is a method in which cups, jars, or wide sections of bamboo are used to create a vacuum and get suctioned to the skin. This suction draws blood to the surface and causes a very superficial bruise. The original idea of this was that the old blood contained toxins that

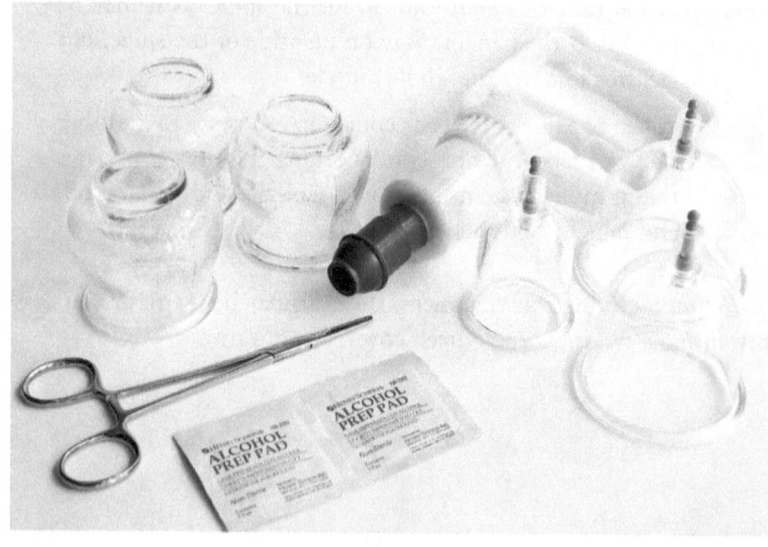

were causing the body to become ill and that pulling the toxin-filled blood out from deeper tissues would allow the toxins to dissipate from the skin. It seems from a modern standpoint that there is some truth to this theory. In the clinic, we use cupping all the time for neck and back pain, as well as for chest colds and congestion. Once again, this seems to be related to increasing blood flow to the affected areas. In this case, the areas would be the entire respiratory system. Remember that bringing fresh blood to the area means that white blood cells are moving in to fight infection. It also means that metabolic waste and inflammation are being carried away from the area.

This may sound uncomfortable, but it feels more like having someone pull the muscles gently from the body. Many patients describe it as if getting a static (non-moving) massage. The sensation should be pleasant, and while helping with cold and flu symptoms, it should also help relax the muscles.

For the sake of keeping things concise, this book will discuss a static technique with both vacuum cups and fire cups. Fire cupping uses glass cups applied with a flame to create a vacuum, and vacuum cupping uses plastic cups and a pump. Both methods are easy to learn and, if done properly, very safe. Cupping sets can be purchased over the Internet, including on eBay. The plastic sets run a bit more but are easier to apply and well worth it for home use. It is difficult, if not impossible, to perform fire cupping on yourself safely, so you will need to recruit someone to perform this on you.

There are some basic rules to follow with cupping:

1. Do not perform any cupping on an open wound, rash, infection site, or other skin problems.

2. If it is uncomfortable, stop and discontinue use.

3. Cupping in one area should normally last about fifteen to twenty minutes, but if very dark bruising is visible after a few minutes, remove the cup.

4. When working on someone with excessive body hair, massage oil can be used to help improve the seal.

5. I've seen cupping done with old mayonnaise jars and tin cans. While this might be effective, the thin lip of these

containers may cut into the skin, so please avoid using them.

6.   Avoid this technique on pregnant women, people who bruise easily, and hemophiliacs.

The plastic set normally comes with several small plastic cups all with a one-way valve at the top and, most importantly, a suction gun. The cups are placed open-side down with the valve facing up. The gun is then placed over the valve and pumped to remove the air. As this is done, the person should feel a mild to moderate pulling sensation. It should never be painful. Depending on the kit, there may be a suggested limit to the number of pumps that should be applied to each cup. If not, it is recommended not to pump more than three times on each cup. To release, press down alongside the cup where it makes contact with the skin. It will break the seal and release the cup.

To get an idea of what the suction-style cups should look like when applied, please see the following picture. Please refer to the cupping location chart under the fire cupping section to see where to apply the cups.

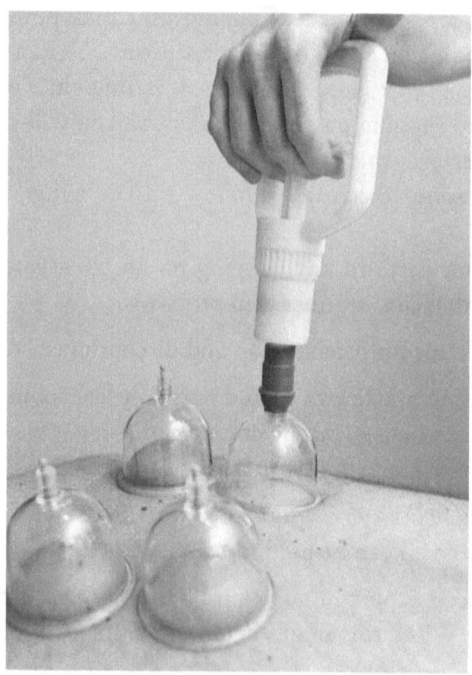

Fire cupping is a bit trickier to apply, but it is more traditional and quite frankly looks "cooler," so many acupuncturists prefer to use this method instead. In addition to the glass cups, you will need hemostats, which are similar to forceps, that will hold a damp alcohol-soaked cotton ball. You will also need a lighter or a lit candle. This method requires a bit of timing as well as a certain level of comfort around an open flame. It is very safe when done properly; that being said, if you don't feel comfortable with this technique, spend the extra money on the plastic cupping set.

For this technique, make sure that there are no flammable materials in or around the work area. You will also need to be working relatively close to the person receiving the cupping, so make sure you can get around the patient comfortably. Have the patient lie down with his or her upper back exposed, and follow closely the steps that follow. For practice, you can try the technique on your leg before working on someone else.

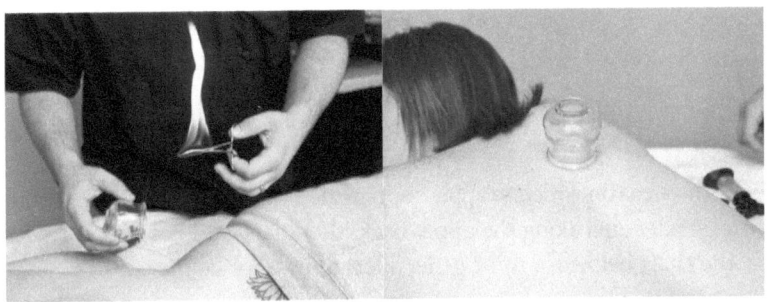

1. Take a cotton ball and lock it in the hemostats. Please make sure they are locked and the cotton ball is secure; this is the reason for most burns associated with cupping.

2. Dip the cotton ball in the rubbing alcohol. The cotton should be wet, but *not dripping.*

3. Light the cotton ball on fire.

4. Pick up a glass cup with the mouth facing down.

5. Standing near, but *not over* the person, swipe the lit cotton ball into the cup quickly and remove it. Do not allow the

cup to get hot from the process. You are only trying to remove the oxygen from the cup.

6.   Quickly place the cup onto the patient's back.

If this technique is done correctly, the cup should pull skin up into it, and the person should feel this pulling. Leave the cups on the skin for up to twenty minutes or until a dark red or purple bruise forms. To remove the cups, press your finger on the skin alongside the cup.

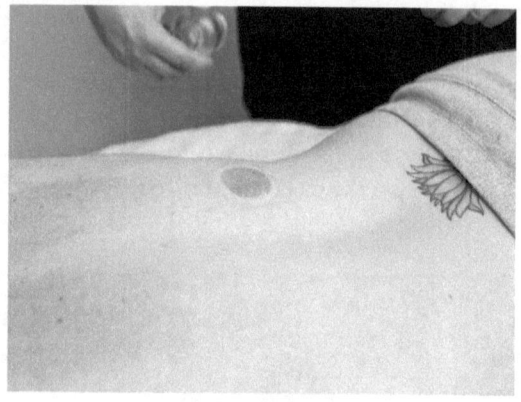

The areas on which to apply cupping do not need to be precise. Think of a broader area along the upper back, shoulders, and neck. Please refer to the chart below for some general locations to place the cups.

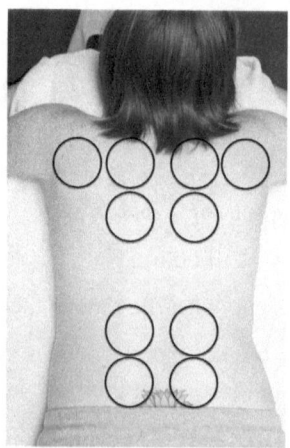

CHAPTER 7
Acupressure and Massage

These next two chapters will focus on acupressure and moxibustion, two techniques that share the same theory of channels and energy as acupuncture. In order to understand how acupressure can help, it is necessary to understand the basics of channel theory from an Oriental medical standpoint. Here is a very basic explanation of channels and acupuncture points and how they work to help you regulate your body functions. The body is covered in unseen pathways called channels or meridians. These channels run up and down the body and have smaller branches that innervate all organs, muscles, and tissues. Along these pathways, energy called qi flows. When a person is feeling ill, the energy in particular areas and channels can become weak or stagnant. When the energy has difficulties flowing, a person starts to show signs of disease. Specific points along the meridians can be stimulated to help correct the flow of energy or help build this energy, which allows the person to recover from a number of conditions, both physical and emotional. The stimulation can occur with needles (called acupuncture), the use of burning herbs (called moxibustion), or acupressure. Acupressure is the stimulation of acupuncture points using manual pressure, normally with your fingers or a blunt massage tool. Acupressure is very safe and can help improve immune system function, relieve sinus pressure, and help achy joints. Feel free to use these points as a standalone therapy or in conjunction with any other therapy we discussed here.

There are thousands of acupuncture points that have developed over the arguably six thousand years that acupuncture has been in existence. This book will cover points that are both easy to locate for the beginner and have the greatest effect on the physical body. You might find that certain points feel more sensitive than others; if so, focus more time on those spots. Sensitivity can be different on points on one side of the body as opposed to the other, which is completely normal. In the descriptions, I will mention when certain points work in conjunction with other points. Pairing these will increase the effect of both points. In general, when searching for the points, find a sore area near the described location and use that sore spot as the acupoint. For convenience, the points will be grouped by symptoms they most strongly address.

To stimulate the point, you can use whichever finger feels comfortable. For most of these points, thumbs or index fingers are usually the easiest and strongest. Pressure should be applied for about twenty to thirty seconds per point. The point should feel a bit sore when pressed, but not painful. Some people may want you to apply constant pressure while others might want to massage the area in a circular motion. This is simply a preference, and you should do whatever feels comfortable to you and the patient.

General Immune System Stimulation:

– St36

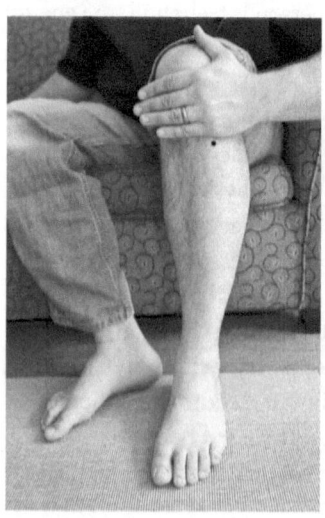

This point was described as the "chicken soup" point by one of my old teachers because of its ability to nourish the body's energy and help the immune system. In classical Chinese medicine terms, this point helps the body take in nutrients from the food we eat and turn it into zhong qi, or central energy, which keeps our body healthy. This central energy feeds out to the surface and builds up our wei qi, or defensive energy. This point is one of the most commonly used points on the body because most of us are either always feeling a little stress or that we could use some more energy. This point has been shown in studies to have many interesting functions after being stimulated. The most important function observed was that white blood cell counts doubled for twenty-four hours after this point was treated; this is a pretty nice immune system boost if you are sick.[9]

This point is located roughly three inches below the lower border of the kneecap, about one finger width away from the shin. Classically this point is located two ways: Place your hand with thumb and index finger making an L around your kneecap so that where the thumb and index meet is situated against the outer lower border of the kneecap. The point will roughly be level with the knuckle of the fifth finger. The second way is to allow your hand to cup the kneecap with fingers pointing downward. The point will be located roughly where your ring finger touches your leg. Make sure your knee is bent at a 90 degree angle when you locate the point with either method. This means sitting up will probably be the easiest way to find it. After finding the point, you can return the leg to whatever position is comfortable.

– Sp6

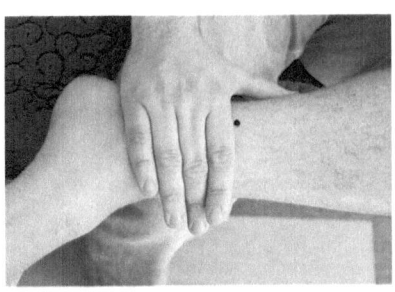

This is another great point to tonify the blood and increase the circulation of qi. It is classically paired with ST 36 and is a crossing point for three of the major channels on the leg. This point is another one that is considered to build up the body to help fight off external pathogens.[10]

This point is located directly above the inside of the ankle roughly where the top of the index finger hits the body when the pinky is placed directly above the inside of the ankle bone (the malleolus) You can locate this point with one leg crossed while sitting up or with your foot flat on the ground.

– LI 11

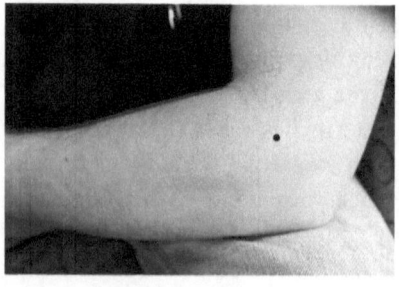

This is another point classically paired with ST36 and is a good point for immune system function as well as sinus issues such as congestion.[11] Classically this point is said to help with fevers, sore throats, and diarrhea, all of which can be commonly found in cold and flu patients.

This point can be located in the depression formed by bending the elbow and following the naturally formed crease to the end. It is located before you get to the outside of the bone in the elbow, but feel free to find the sorest point in the area and use that for acupressure. After finding the sore point you can relax the arm.

Sinus Congestion and Headaches

– LV3

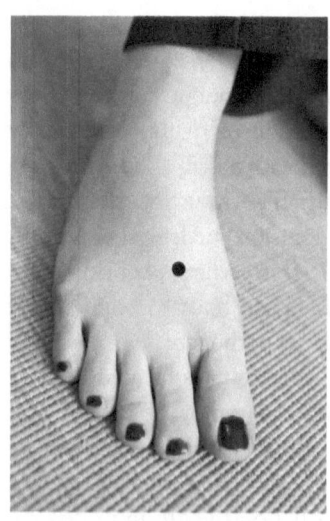

This point is one of the big guns for headaches, especially headaches that affect the temples and side of the head. It is said to open the channels and can be used to treat congestion, headaches, dizziness, and swelling in the eyes. The LV3 point is very often used with the next point, LI4, for a big qi moving and clearing effect.[12]

This point is located on the top of the foot between the bones leading to the first and second toes. To find the point, slide your fingers toward the ankle starting at the web between the first and second toes. The point should be where the two long bones in the foot (the metatarsals) meet. Look for the most sensitive spot and apply pressure there.

– LI 4

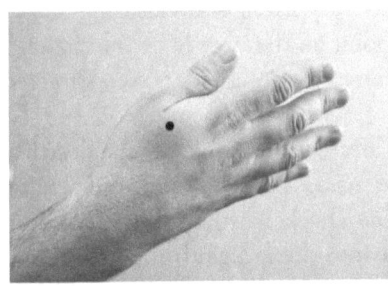

This point is known as the command point for the head and face. It can be used to treat any condition involving the head, eyes, mouth, and sinuses, making it particularly useful for cold and flu symptoms. Paired with LV3, this group of points is known as the four gates[13] and can be used for any head condition as well as for pain throughout the body.

This point is located between the thumb and index finger on the high point of the muscle. Some people may locate this point at the end of the crease formed when the thumb is pulled next to the rest of the hand. Use this as a starting area and feel around for the most sensitive spot. Press toward the bone or pinch the tissue between your thumb and index finger, depending on which method is more sensitive.

– Du23

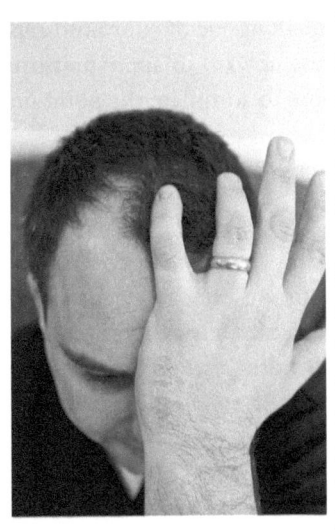

This point has a strong effect on the frontal sinuses and can also be used to help with headaches. The name of this point is *spirit garden* and is often used when there are no cold and flu symptoms, to help with sleep issues.

This point is located about an inch into the hairline, straight up from the nose. It can be found easily by placing the heel of the palm against the bridge of the nose so that the fifth finger lines up with the bridge. The point should lie roughly under the tip of the pinky and there should also be a slight indentation. If active, the point should feel sore and slightly spongy. Once you locate it with the pinky finger, feel free to switch to another finger so it is more comfortable to stimulate this point.

– LI20

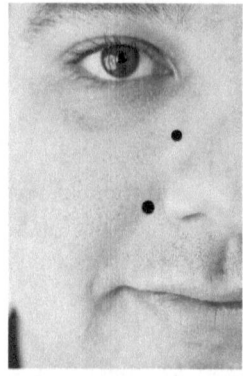

This is another very strong sinus clearing point. It is the last point on the large intestine channel and can be paired with LI4 for an even stronger effect.

LI 20 is located to the sides of the nostrils, between the nasal passages and the crease formed by the cheek when smiling. You can press straight into the face with this point, but to help physically open the sinuses, press in and pull away from the nose. [14]

– Bi Tong

Bi Tong literally means nose pain. In clinic, many acupuncturists will needle LI 20 and aim the needle toward this point.[15] It is another point that is commonly used for sinus congestion, and it is roughly the area that is pulled open by certain breathing strips worn by athletes and snorers.

To find this point, slide your finger up alongside of your nose and stop when you feel the bone. You can press upward to apply pressure to this point or pinch the bridge of the nose to stimulate the point on both sides of the nose at once.

– GB20

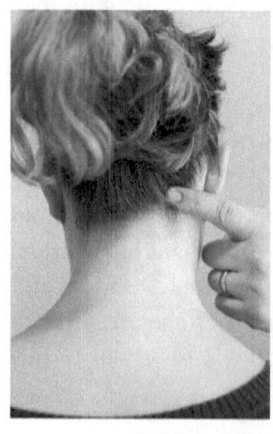

This is another big point that covers lots of different conditions. It can be used for headaches, puffy eyes, sinus congestion, sore throat, and runny nose. It strongly affects the brain and sense organs, so it is great to use for head colds and flu symptoms.

This point can be located by making an L with your thumb and index finger and placing it at the front border of your ear. Allow the thumb to wrap around the bottom of the skull. This point should be located under the thumbpad in a depression just below the base of the skull. To stimulate GB20, you can apply pressure with your thumbs directly into the neck or slightly upward toward the bone.[16]

Fever/Chills:

In Oriental medical theory, the back of the neck is a place where external pathogens can enter the body and cause disease.[17] One of these pathogenic factors is considered to be the wind. Wind blowing on the neck is thought to be one of the causes of diseases like the cold and flu. It is believed that this area acts like a shortcut to the deeper tissues of the body. In most Asian cultures, you may see people wearing scarves during the winter and lighter scarves in the spring and fall. They are protecting this sensitive area from invading pathogens in order to keep disease away. These next three points all have the function to open up the back of the neck to let out any pathogens that may have gotten in the body and cause disease. A folk-style cold remedy is to pinch the back of the neck from the base of the skull to the shoulders, lightly and repeatedly, until the area comes up red. This is similar to the Gua Sha technique previously discussed in chapter 5.

– Du14

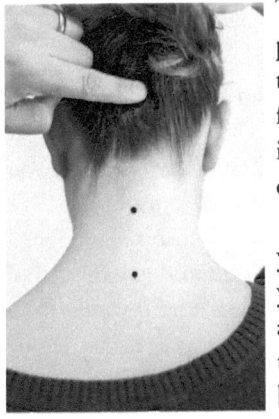

This point is a major point for expelling pathogenic wind from the body.[18] It is great to use for neck stiffness as well as chills and fevers, and because of its ease of location, it's also ideal for moxibustion, which will be discussed in the next chapter.

Du14 can be found by following along your shoulders to the midline of the base of your neck. Keep level with your shoulder and do not follow the upward curve of your trapezius muscles. The name of this point is big bone, and it is located in the space below the seventh cervical vertebrae, which in most people sticks out the farthest in the neck. Stimulating this point can be done by pressing into the body toward the front in between the vertebra or by pinching the skin.

– *Du16*

This point is called wind mansion, indicating that this is truly a place where the pathogen can blow into the body and build up quite a stronghold. Stimulation of this point can help loosen the foundation of the mansion and hopefully evict the illness.

This point is very easy to locate. Simply feel along the base of the skull around the midline of the back of your head. You should feel a bump, which is called the External Occipital Protuberance. Du 16 is located directly below that bump and can be stimulated by pressing in or by pinching the area of the skin.

– *Du15*

This point is found in between the previous two points and has a very similar effect. It is used for conditions that affect the throat, sinuses, and neck. It has the function of releasing all types of external pathogens.

It can be located by placing the fingers of one hand along the back of the neck without using the thumb. The pinky should be level with the hairline. The middle finger should fall very close to the space between two of the cervical vertebra; the point is located in that space. If you are having problems locating the point, tilt your head up and the point should be where the back of the neck creases the most.

Immune Enhancing Protocol

The following is a simple immune tonic treatment that can be used before symptoms set in, or just when you feel run down. Of course, when you get sick, you can turn to these points to shorten the duration of the illness. You can stimulate the points on both sides of the body for a stronger effect. This treatment is based on a dozen similar acupuncture protocols all designed to boost qi and blood and stimulate white blood cell production.[19] All of these points have been discussed in previous chapters, and if you wish to add other points into this protocol, feel free.

- Du23
- LI11
- ST 36
- LI4
- LV3

CHAPTER 8
Moxibustion: Healing with Heat

Moxibustion is considered by many acupuncturists to be the other half of acupuncture. In fact, the two characters that make up the Chinese term for acupuncture are a hand inserting a needle (zheng) and a smoldering herb (jiu). Classically, acupuncture and moxibustion always had a very close relationship.[20] In fact, one of the classical acupuncture sayings goes, "If all else fails, try moxibustion."

So exactly what is moxibustion, also called moxa? Moxa is made from the herb commonly known as mugwort (*artemesia vulgaris* and other species). This plant grows all over the world and is very common in mountain valleys. The herb is dried out, crushed up, and the darker green plant material is separated from a light, fluffy, wool-like material, which will eventually be used for moxibustion. The moxa "wool" is dried for three years to get a finished product. There are several grades of moxa based on how well the dense plant material is separated from the wool-like substance. The higher the grade of moxa, the lighter in color it is and in general it can be burned closer if not directly on the skin.

A note about the general smell of moxa

Often times, patients will come into an acupuncture clinic wondering why it smells of marijuana. It is not pot; it is the smell of moxibustion. Depending on the quality of moxa, that odd odor may be very strong, or virtually non-existent. Most people find the odor pleasant, but some really do not like it at all. If you have roommates, or neighbors who may object to the smell, you may want to explain to them what you are doing prior to performing these techniques. If you don't want the smell at all you can try using smokeless versions of all the techniques this chapter will discuss. In general, the smokeless products produce very little smoke and smell more like a freshly lit grill rather than an illegal herb. The smokeless versions may be a better alternative for some. However, they tend to burn at a higher temperature, are harder to light, and it is debated whether or not you still get the effect of the herbal properties from the smokeless versions.

Moxibustion has several amazing effects on the body, all of which promote proper blood flow, red and white blood cell production, and systemic healing. It has even been linked to longevity in some modern studies.[21] Many old acupuncturists throughout history attest to this function.

It can be used locally on points, but it can also be used to add heat to a general area. Why would people do moxibustion instead of acupressure? Moxibustion is used mainly to get a different stimulation than just pressure. When moxa is burned, it emits an infrared light that has been shown to help produce energy on a cellular level. The heat also helps increase circulation locally and systemically. The herb and the resin have been shown to be antifungal, antibacterial, and, most important for treating colds and flus, antiviral.

As moxibustion involves smoldering herbs and fire, this book will be discussing the safest methods of moxibustion, but by no means will it discuss all of them. This book is intended to help people treat themselves when they are not feeling well, not land them in a burn ward. So, as a secondary disclaimer, do not try to tolerate more heat, do not burn moxa directly on the skin, and do not attempt one of these techniques if you are uncomfortable doing so.

Now that that is out of the way, moxibustion can be performed safely and effectively at home, but it will require you to purchase a few items, preferably before you get sick. These styles of moxibustion are extremely safe and moxa, like fine wine, is said to get better with age, so ordering moxa and keeping the moxa in the back of your closet until you need it isn't a bad idea. You may be able to find many of these items on eBay. If not, you may have to search for an acupuncture supply store. Some acupuncture supply stores may not sell to you directly, but they might refer you to a local acupuncturist who will. When purchasing supplies, ask the acupuncturist to show you the techniques you've read in this book to ensure that you are performing them correctly.

There are literally hundreds of methods and devices used to apply moxibustion to the body safely. Over the centuries, all sorts of devices have been used, and with the development of heat-tolerant plastics and silicone, it seems like more moxibustion tools are being rolled out every year. That taken into account, there is no way a small novice-friendly book could possibly cover the entire scope and breadth of moxibustion. The goal here is to show the simplest and safest methods to stimulate the body using moxibustion. As such, this book will cover three very easy and safe methods of moxibustion. Those methods are:

- using the Korean Bong Rae moxa ring
- using a moxa pole
- using stick-on moxa cones

As a general cautionary note, all of these moxibustion techniques should feel warm, not hot. Always err on the side of caution with moxibustion techniques and do not get burned.

In this section, we will be using some of the points used in the acupressure section as well as some additional points and areas depending on the moxibustion device used. As a general note, there are some points on the head and face that can be used with moxibustion, but it requires a style of moxibustion not covered in this book and it is best to leave that to a professional acupuncturist. Please do not try home moxibustion on these points: Du23, Du16, GB20, LI20, Bi Tong.

Bong Rae Moxa Bowl

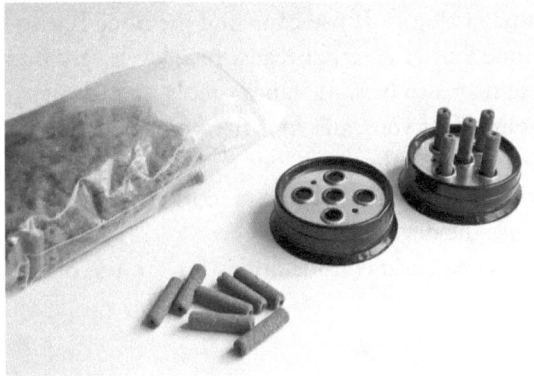

Bong Rae Moxa is probably one of the easiest moxibustion methods available today. It is designed to keep from getting too hot as well as to cover a relatively large area instead of having to worry about being directly over small acupuncture points. Sometimes people refer to the Bong Rae moxa device as a bowl or a ring, and most places that sell them or use them will use the terms interchangeably, so don't worry if the place selling it describes it as a ring instead of a bowl. Bong Rae comes in two sizes: a large rubber ring that has five holes for hard-pressed moxa "plugs," and a small rubber ring that holds only one hole. As the intended use for this style of moxa is to cover a larger area, the larger ring will be used in this book.

There are several advantages to this style of moxibustion for the home user. We have already mentioned the mild heat and the ability to cover a larger area, which will keep burns to a minimum. Several other benefits include cost; both the plugs and the ring are relatively cheap. The tools are durable; steel and rubber allow for a long life. They are easy to use; simply put, you can "plug" them in and light them and you are ready to go. One of my favorite things about this device is that it not only focuses on delivering a safe heat to the body, but by design it produces a heavy smoky resin that is funneled down to the skin via the holes in the moxa plugs themselves. This resin also has immune-enhancing properties and can be left on for a couple hours after use or wiped off. Note that the resin will look a little like a spray-on tan, but while it will wash off your body completely, it will stain clothes, so if you wish to leave the resin on for a while, you should cover it with some gauze and tape.

There are quite a few other similar devices for what is called "indirect moxibustion."[22] If you can't find the Bong Rae style, you can try another one, but be careful because heat levels vary from device to device. There may also be some fancier tools that require you to press the moxa yourself. If you can't find the Bong Rae and would like to try one of the many other tools out there, please contact a licensed acupuncturist or Oriental medicine practitioner and have them show you how to use the device.

Here are some basic considerations for the use of the Bong Rae Moxa ring:

1. As with any type of moxa, remember you are working with something that is burning. Have a bowl with water or an ashtray nearby to extinguish the moxa.

2. Some heat is good, but burning yourself is not. Keep the heat levels comfortable. *Do not* tough it out.

3. Make sure the moxa plugs are inserted into the holes well. If they are loose or broken, do not use them.

4. The plugs should be in the ring prior to lighting them.

5. The plugs do take some time to light; use a candle or a strong butane cigar lighter and make sure they are well lit.

6. You do not need to put a moxa plug in every open space. If the heat is too much with five plugs, try using only three.

7. Make sure the ring can sit on your body and be stable. The rubber should be in full contact with your body.

8. Feel free to reload the ring after all the plugs have burned down. You can keep going over areas as long as they don't feel too hot.

As mentioned before, this device provides heat to a broad area, so we will be discussing its use on the abdomen and back.

Bong Rae on the Abdomen

According to Oriental Medical theory, the abdomen is the area where the qi and blood are produced and then circulated to keep us healthy. A large portion of immune system function is now shown to occur in our intestines, which is why there are so many ads for yogurt with live bacteria and other products to help restore a healthy intestinal flora. Interestingly, in Oriental medicine, it is said that the lungs and large intestine are paired organs. When we treat the large intestine, we can help improve lung function, which definitely will be of great benefit to someone with a cold. Also, when treating the abdomen, we help improve digestion, which allows your body to get the nutrients it needs to help recover, as well as helping produce more white blood cells to fight off infections.

The Bong Rae Bowl can be placed anywhere on the abdomen and slowly moved around. There is no need to keep to strict locations, but look at the photo for some particularly good areas to focus on.

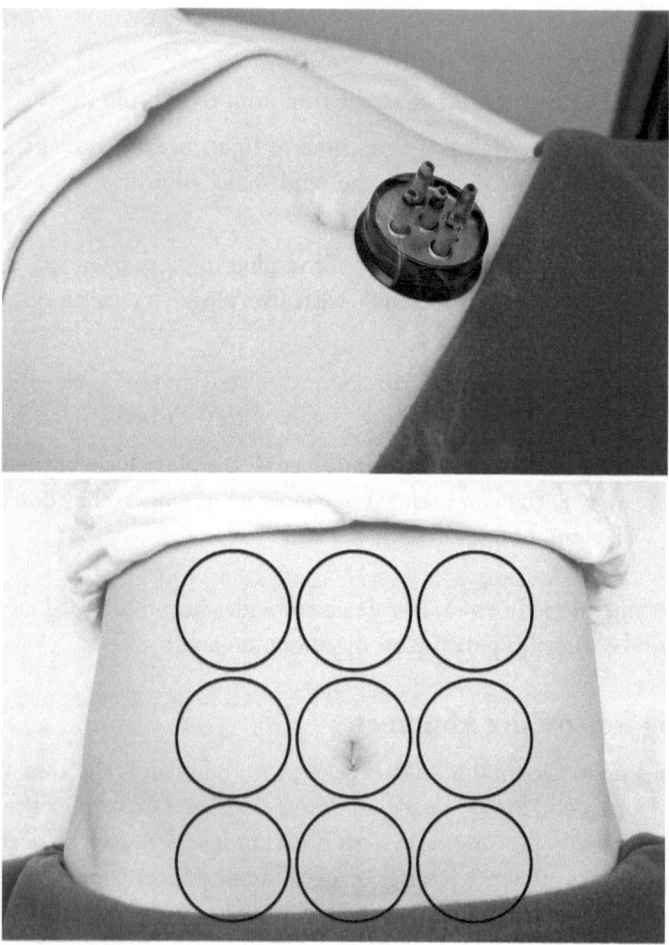

Note that there are five spots, with the center being the belly button. Basically, you or someone helping you can move the moxa ring straight to the left and right of the navel as well as directly above and below it. These areas of the abdomen correspond very closely with both digestion and immune system function, but you can also move the ring diagonally to make a nine-circle box. You should move the ring if it gets too hot, but it may burn out before that happens, at which point you can refill and light it and move it to the next spot.

Bong Rae Bowl For Back Treatments

When cold and flu symptoms cause tightness in the chest, coughing, chest congestion, and back stiffness, this type of moxibustion can really help. For this technique, you will need someone to help you. The moxa bowl must be placed on the back, and because you have no easy access to it, the person must stay with you the whole time the moxa is burning and will be the person moving the bowl around the back. In general, anywhere the moxa ring can lay on the back where it is completely stable, you can place it. Be careful of people who have excess curvature in their upper or lower backs. You do not want the moxa ring to tip over. For coughing, congestion, chest tightness, and respiratory issues, try burning the moxa ring between the two shoulder blades. You can slowly move it in a line alongside the spine, waiting for each area to get comfortably warm or covered with the resin. With digestive issues, place the ring along the spine in the area just below where the rib cage ends. For lower back tightness, you can place the rings along the spine right above the hips.

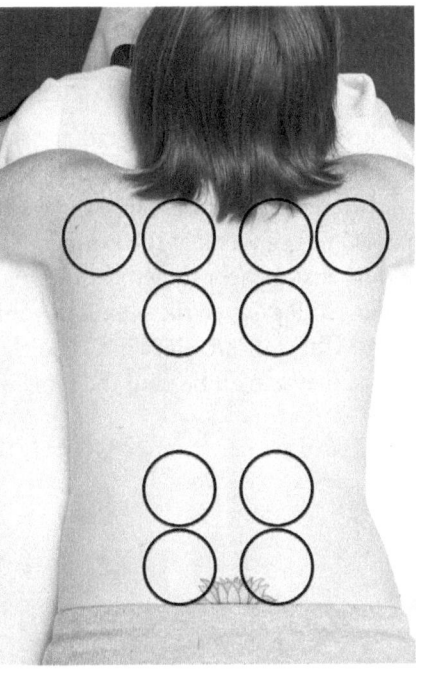

Moxa Poles

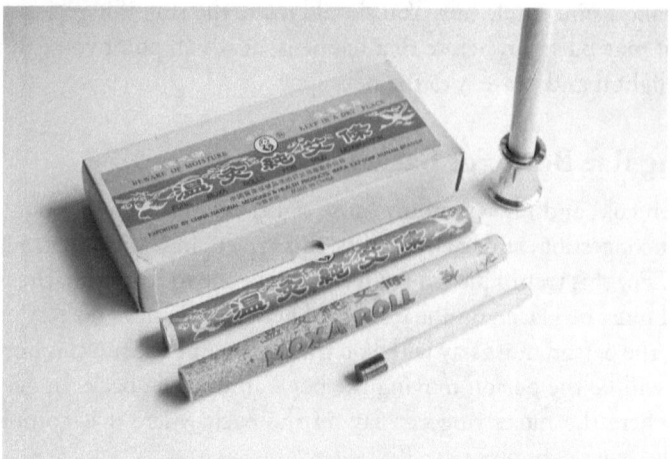

The traditional moxa pole can be used to warm a specific point or an entire area of the body; it is one of the oldest methods of moxibustion and is also one of the simplest. Moxa poles are basically a cigar made with mugwort and paper rather than tobacco, but these are not to smoke! Some moxa poles have an outer wrapper that must be peeled off before lighting while others have the label printed on the burnable paper. You can look at the moxa pole, and if there is a thin paper with a thicker rice paper underneath, chances are the outer paper should be removed. Please see the photo for some of the different types of moxa poles. They all are similar, and although some may add additional herbs, they can all be used the same way.

General Technique Tips for the Moxa Pole

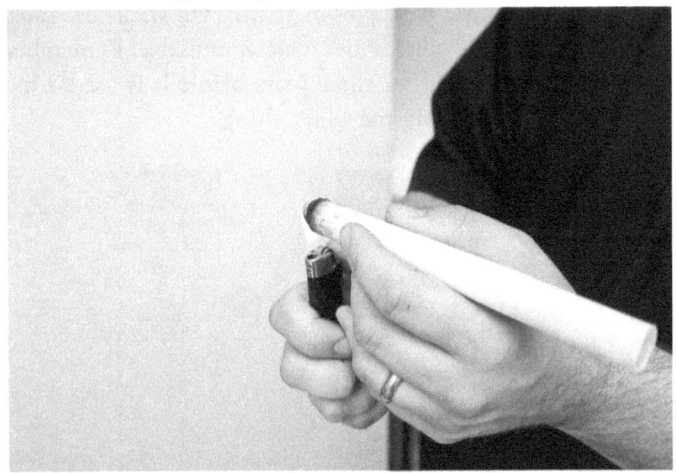

- To use the moxa pole, light the end on fire and give it a few seconds to develop a nice red ember.

- Use your other hand as a heat-sensing hand, and always keep it in contact with the area being heated. If your heat sensing hand is too hot, the body part underneath it is too hot! If you have a friend doing this technique on you, have them use their hand to sense the heat as well.

- Keep an ashtray or cup of water nearby; when the ash builds up on the moxa pole, knock it off as you would ash a cigar.

- To put the moxa stick out, either cut the burning part off with a very sharp knife on a non-flammable surface or keep a small jar of salt or sand on hand. Simply put the lit end of the pole into the sand or salt, and it will extinguish itself quickly. You can buy fancy metal moxa pole extinguishers, but unless you are using the moxa pole often, it may not be worth it, as the sand or salt works very well. The advantages of the sand or salt method are that you don't have to cut something that is burning (you just put it in the sand or salt), and there is an even bigger bonus: when you extinguish the moxa in sand or salt you form a nice point like a pen when you light the pole again.

Whatever you do, do not extinguish the moxa pole in water. The moxa is so porous that it will wick the water up the pole very quickly and make it unusable. Remember that moxa is dried for three years before it is used. One quick dip could ruin the whole thing.

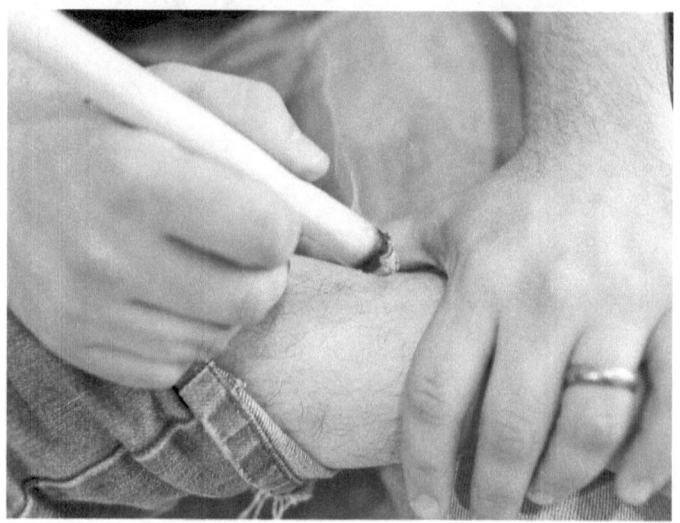

Instructions for stimulating points with the moxa pole:

- Light the moxa pole at one end; allow it to get evenly red across the tip. Knock off excess ash as it builds up into an ashtray or cup of water.

- Place your heat-sensing hand near the point to get moxa. Keep this hand in a C or an L shape as it rests against the skin. If you have someone doing this technique on you, he or she should use his or her free hand in the same manner. If he or she feels that the moxa is too hot, he or she should pull it away from you.

- The moxa pole should be held a few inches away until the point or heat-sensing hand feels comfortably warm.

- Pull the moxa away from the point and allow the area to cool off for a few seconds.

• The moxa pole can then be brought back a few more times. Classically, acupuncturists would do this three, five, or nine times based on Chinese numerology, but you can do it until the point feels warm to the touch. Use the points listed in the acupressure section, minus the points on the face or head. A good overall treatment would be the immune system treatment minus Du 23, which would be LI11, St36, LI4, and LV3. Remember that because the heat from the moxa radiates, exact point location is not as important. Even if you are close, the heat will still have a positive effect on the point.

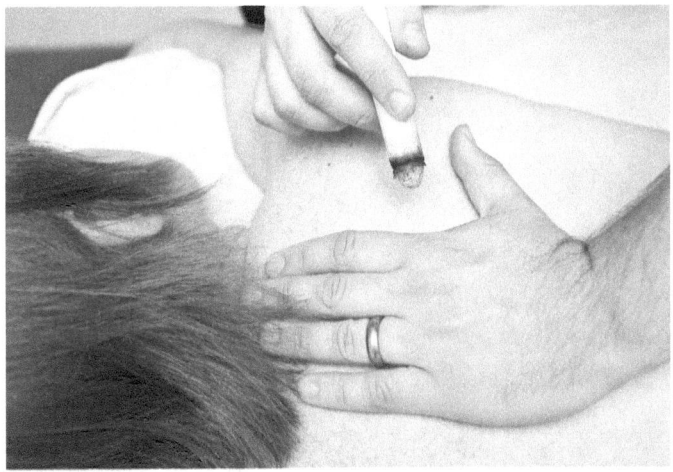

You can also use pole moxa to "paint" heat in an area of the body. This is a great way to help with general soreness, chest congestion, and chills. This technique will require a partner.

General steps to paint an area using the moxa pole

• Light the moxa pole the same way as before.

• Have the person performing the technique still keep his hand on the body.

• Determine where on the body you wish to be covered with heat. Good suggestions would be the neck and shoulders, the abdomen, or the lower back.

- Keep the moxa pole: moving up and down the area of the body as if the heat is being painted on. Use slow, sweeping strokes until the area feels evenly warm. It is important to keep the heat-sensing hand in contact with the body close to the hot end of the moxa pole. When doing this technique, try to keep the moxa moving at a steady pace and keep it an even distance from the surface of the skin. This will allow the body to be heated evenly and keep the risk of burns to a minimum.

Stick-On Moxa

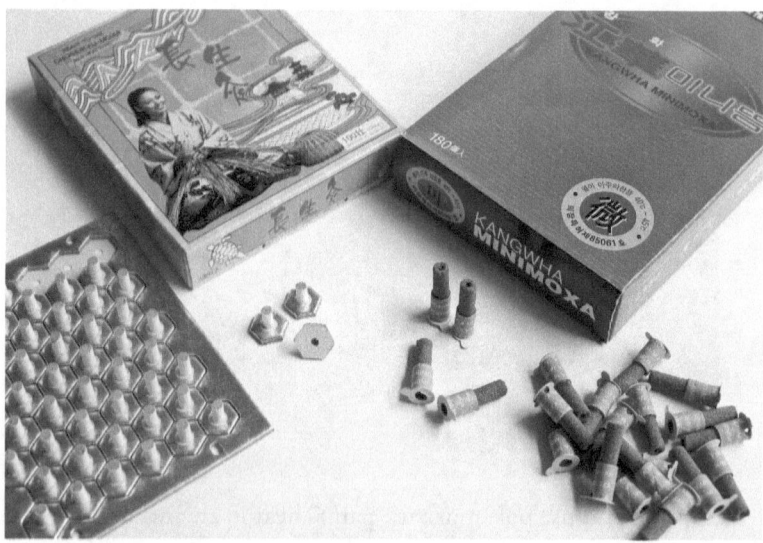

Stick-on moxa are manufactured by several companies and all have their own unique appearance and heat levels. Fortunately, they all have a very similar design and method of use. In general, stick-on moxa is made of a pressed or rolled moxa cone with a cardboard base. The bottom of the base has a mild adhesive to allow the moxa to stick on to the acupuncture point. The cardboard keeps the moxa far enough away from the skin to provide mild warming without causing a burn; however, when burning multiple stick-on moxa cones on a site, be sure to check the skin between each one so that burns are avoided.

The same point restrictions apply for this type of moxa as the pole moxa: no points on the face, hairline, or head. As previously stated, all of the stick-on moxa brands have varying heat levels; some come with a pad that goes between the skin and the moxa to make the heat even milder. It's a good idea to try using one or two of them on an area that you can get to easily until you have a feel for how hot that particular style gets. If they get too hot as they burn down, remove them earlier rather than attempting to tough it out. Remember, don't get burned! With this technique, you may want to have a set of tweezers nearby to remove moxa cones as they burn down. You should also have either a small bowl of water or ashtray to dispose of the used moxa.

The actual technique for stick-on moxa is relatively simple.

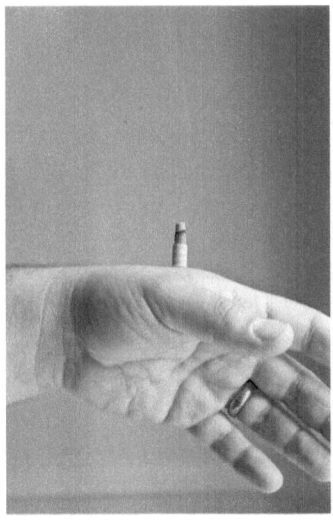

1. Locate the acupuncture point and use any of the non-head and face points from the acupressure. When doing this technique, find a comfortable position where you or a partner can easily access the point to receive moxa.

2. Remove the wax paper backing from the stick-on moxa, or remove the stick-on moxa from the board of moxa, depending on which style you use.

3. Light the top of the stick-on moxa with a lighter or candle. If you are using the hard-pressed moxa style, it may take some time for the whole tip to light.

4. Place the sticky backing to the acupuncture point. Make sure that it is solid enough before moving your hand away. At this point, try to remain in one position—movement might make the moxa fall.

5. Allow the moxa to burn down. As it burns, it should get warmer. If it feels too hot, take it off. Remember that level and remove the next round prior to it burning that low.

6. Repeat steps 1–5 multiple times. Remember, classically, we use odd numbered times, with three, five, and nine being the best.

With this technique, the immune-enhancing protocol can be even more immune-enhancing, just remember to omit Du 23. You can treat each point once and then repeat the cycle again and again to get to three, five, or nine rounds, or you can do each point three, five, or nine times before moving to the next spot.

CHAPTER 9
Closing

When we are sick, it seems like it takes forever to recover. Not only are our symptoms miserable, but even the most common activities take longer and only seem to drain us more. Hopefully, the techniques in this book will help you recover more quickly. It may be a good idea for you to get some of the items you need for these techniques and try them prior to getting ill. You will be more comfortable performing them, and that will be helpful when it comes time to use them when you are sick. These treatments will all be most beneficial at the initial onset of colds and flus, so at the first sign of sniffles, sneezes, cough, congestion, or fever, give some of these treatments a try. If you are unsure about any of these techniques, please contact your local acupuncturist or go to my website: www.tryacu.com.

Be well.

ABOUT THE AUTHOR

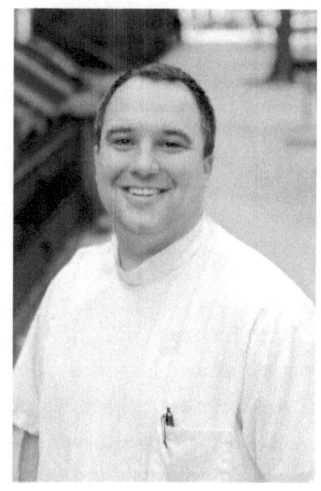

Tom Ingegno, MSOM, LAc is a licensed acupuncturist and certified animal acupuncturist with over a decade of experience in Oriental medicine. He has a master's degree in Oriental medicine and a bachelor's degree in professional health science. Tom is nationally certified (NCCAOM) and licensed in both New York and Maryland. He has been studying internal cultivation arts, including meditation, qigong, xingyi, and tai chi, since 1995. Tom has also been formally trained in Chinese herbal medicine.

He has taught at the New York College of Health Professions and the Pacific College of Oriental Medicine in New York. Tom was a board member of Edo Kai Traditional Acupuncture Society and has been published in several different issues of *North American Journal of Oriental Medicine* (NAJOM) as well as consumer magazines and websites. He has treated FEMA rescue workers for both pain and emotional stress during the New York 9/11 rescue effort. He has also lectured about acupuncture and men's health at Baltimore's City Hall as part of Baltimore's TV25 program on Men in Science and several Johns Hopkins groups. In 2010, Tom Ingegno was voted Best Acupuncturist by *Baltimore City Paper*'s readers' poll.

He is also certified to treat companion animals, including dogs, cats, and horses. He volunteers to treat animals with several Baltimore rescues and has been a consultant at the Maryland Zoo in Baltimore. Tom has performed acupuncture on a pit bull rescued from Michael Vick, camels in Egypt, and a giraffe at the Maryland Zoo in Baltimore.

Tom continues lecturing about acupuncture and Oriental medicine and studying with prominent acupuncturists both in the US and abroad to ensure that he continues to expand his knowledge base and skills to provide the best possible care for all sentient beings.

ENDNOTES

1. Gil Marks, *Encyclopedia of Jewish Food* (New Jersey: John Wiley and Sons, 2010), 119.

2. Peter C K Cheung, *Mushrooms as Functional Foods* (New Jersey: John Wiley and Sons 2008).

3. Lizzie Collingham, *A Tale of Cooks and Conquerers,* (New York: Oxford University Press, 2006), 187–214.

4. Carl-Herman Hempen Toni Fischer, *A materia medica for Chinese medicine: plants, minerals, and animal products,* (Munich: Elsevier Health Sciences, 2009), 122.

5. Stefan Chmelik, *Chinese Herbal Secrets: The Key to Total Health,* (Garden City Park: Penguin, 1999).

6. Joseph P. Hou and Youyu Jin, *The Healing Power of Chinese herbs and medicinal recipes,* (Routledge, 2005), 303.

7. Michael Tierra and Lesley Tierra, *Chinese Traditional Herbal Medicine Vol. II Materia Medica & Herbal Resource,* (Twin Lakes: Lotus Press, 1998).

8. James Kedzie Sayre, *Ancient Herbs and Modern Herbs: a comprehensive reference guide to medicinal herbs, human ailments and possible herbal remedies,* (Bottlebrush Press, 2001), 151.

9. Subhuti Dharmandanda PhD, "Zusanli (Stomach 36)", *Institute for Traditional Medicine,* http://www.itmonline. org/acupuncture.htm

10. Chris Jarmey and Llaira Bouratinos, *A Practical Guide to Acu-Points,* (Berkley: North Atlantic Books, 2008), 123.

11. Jarmey and Bouratinos, *A Practical Guide to Acu-Points,* 69.

12. Bob Flaws, *Curing Headaches Naturally with Chinese Medicine,* (Boulder: Blue Poppy Enterprises Inc, 1999), 79.

13. Flaws, *Curing Headaches Naturally with Chinese Medicine,* 79.

14. Jarmey and Bouratinos, *A Practical Guide to Acu-Points,* 75.

15. Jarmey and Bouratinos, *A Practical Guide to Acu-Points,* 326.

16. Michael Reed Gach, *Acupressure's Potent Points: A Guide to Self-Care for Common Ailments,* (New York: Bantam Books, 1990), 60–62.

17. Tina Sohn and Robert C Sohn, *Amma Therapy: a complete textbook of Oriental bodywork and medical principles,* (Rochester: Inner Traditions / Bear and Company, 1997), 297.

18. Peter Deadman, Mazin Al-Khafaji and Keven Baker, *A Manual of Acupuncture,* (East Sussex: Journal of Chinese Medicine Publications, 1998).

19. Jeremy Ross, *Acupuncture point combinations:the key to clinical success,* (Elsevier Health Sciences, 1995).

20. Xiaofei, Jianhua Mu, *Acupuncture and Moxibustion,* IOS Press, 2000.

21. Honora Lee Wolfe "Moxibustion for longevity and health preservation", *Townsend Letter for Doctors and Patients,* FindArticles.com. 09 Apr, 2011. http://findarticles.com/p/articles/mi_m0ISW/is_269/ai_n15986339/

22. Andrew Ellis, Nigel Wiseman, and Ken Boss, *Fundamentals of Chinese Acupuncture,* (Taos: Paradigm Publications, 1991), 24.